Growing an Internal Garden to Cope With

Chronic Pain, Illness, and Depression

Renee Alter

www.reneealter.com
www.reneealtersatmosphere.com
www.amazon.com/author/reneealter
www.facebook.com/reneealtersatmosphere

Revised 6/19/2020

This little book includes a narrowed down summary of what I learned in my personal journey through chronic pain, illness, and depression. Life is a journey, not a destination. I am still on the journey, writing new blog posts as well as updating my website and Pinterest with new links to articles and videos I find. You can find them here:

www.reneealtersatmosphere.com

pinterest.com/reneealter

If, after you use this book, you would like to delve deeper into your healing journey, I can refer you to the practitioners who have been assisting me. You can contact me through my website/blog (the above link). There is a contact form in the right column. From a cell phone, scroll to the bottom and click on View Web Version.

Table of Contents

Introduction

Chronic illness and/or pain of any kind can seem like it is stripping your life away. It does. It affects the relationships you have with your family and friends. It affects your ability to work. It strips you of whatever identity you formed through your work and relationships. Financial hardship soon follows. Life becomes stressful… leaving you stuck in fight or flight. If you experienced trauma as a child (most people do), it has lasting affects your brain and nervous system. Stress affects your digestion and your immune system. You lose your ability to cope. Severe depression follows. It affects your ability to take care of yourself, so you end up being dependent on others… others who have no understanding or compassion for what you are dealing with. It flat out sucks. I know.

Because you are in pain, you stop moving or you move much slower. The less you move, the worse the pain seems to get. When you don't move 'it,' you lose 'it' – your physical strength and your ability to feel good emotionally. When you stop breathing deeply, your body does not get enough oxygen and does not eliminate enough toxins, again intensifying pain. Pain makes your muscles tense up, which causes more pain.

I started out with many years of chronic fatigue syndrome after a bout with mono when I was 18. I was sick for six months before it was diagnosed. I didn't know how to process all the trauma I had been through. Antibiotics had destroyed my gut, so I developed food sensitivities. Add to this the neck injury while doing a head stand and two car accidents, one of which I sustained a nasty whiplash. Plus, I was born with spina bifida occulta and developed spondylolisthesis at L5-S1 with a bilateral pars fracture. Basically, my spine is slipped halfway off my sacrum... which was not diagnosed until I was almost 50. What I was diagnosed with is fibromyalgia and carpal tunnel syndrome.

I was finally able to recover from CFS after finding a doctor of Natural Medicine, and even so, it took two years. While I was on the treatment program, I began to listen to Louise Hay's tapes on *You Can Heal Your Life*, and as I learned to love myself more and improve my mental health, illness seemed to disappear and the amount of pain I was in decreased. I learned to change the relationship I have with pain and do a lot more work in the self-love department. I learned that FMS is what I have, not who I am. I learned that finding a purpose in life (writing books and helping other aspiring authors write theirs) raised my mood which increased my ability to cope.

Maybe you were told the pain in your body is all in your head. When I was told this, I got angry. It was years before I learned that your thoughts, emotions, and your perceptions can intensify the sensations of pain. When you include one or more thinking errors, you can end up wallowing in self-pity. Then no one seems to want to be around you, so all your friendships disappear. You find yourself overwhelmed by intense neediness. Your self-esteem is deeply affected especially when others invalidate what you are going through. There will also be GRIEF for the parts of your life you have lost, which will be as intense as the death of someone you love. Everything is interconnected.

Most likely, you were or will be offered antidepressants which can trigger even more anger as you shout silently to the world that no one understands – that it is not all in your head! The pain is REAL! Antidepressants are being given in attempts to shift brain chemistry so you will produce more serotonin and norepinephrine which ultimately reduces pain. But be cautious. Sometimes (like in my case) you can have bad reactions to them, including feeling suicidal. What they say in the commercials about Cymbalta, happened to me. I recommend that if you accept an anti-depressant of any kind that you start with ½ of the lowest dose and gradually increase until you begin to feel relief. And hopefully, you won't need to take them for the rest of your life. However, Dr. John Bergman (the chiropractor my family members who live in California go to) teaches that serotonin is made in your gut, and that your gut will produce it when you make it healthy again.

It is important that you create a healthcare team that includes alternatives beyond just medical and medication. These practitioners should include one or more of the following: a good chiropractor (ask around to find out who other people with your similar condition go to and whether they are satisfied), a doctor of Natural Medicine that will work with your entire body vs. a small part of it, a nutritionist (you ARE what you EAT), a massage therapist (touch is healing), acupuncture, reflexology, Reiki and or sound practitioner (our bodies are made up of energy), biofeedback, neurofeedback, or a hypnotherapist (who can teach you how to mindfully / mentally change pain sensations or help you to stop smoking), a physical therapist and or personal trainer (who can teach you how to use the muscles you still have properly), a motivational coach or practitioner of positive psychology (to help you focus on the positive).

There is a huge difference between how you deal with pain/illness/depression when you feel helpless, powerless, and depressed and when you have serenity. The goal I have for you (and for myself) is summarized by this version of The Serenity Prayer I found:

Serenity Prayer

God grant me the serenity...

Serenity means that I no longer recoil from the past, live in jeopardy because of my present behavior, or worry about the unknown future. I seek regular times to re-create myself and I avoid those times of depletion that make me vulnerable to despair and to old self-destructive patterns.

...to accept the things I cannot change...

Accepting change means that I do not cause suffering for myself by clinging to that which no longer exists. All that I can count on is that nothing will be stable—except how I respond to the transforming cycles in my life of birth, growth, and death.

...the courage to change the things I can...

Giving up my attempts to control outcomes does not require that I give up my boundaries or my best efforts. It does mean my most honest appraisal of the limits of what I can do.

...and the wisdom to know the difference.

Wisdom becomes the never forgotten recognition of all those times when it seemed there was no way out, and new paths opened up like miracles in my life.

You Are Made Up of Body, Mind, and Spirit

Your body is quite miraculous. You are an amazing Universe of over 70 trillion cells! There are videos on YouTube that document perfect creation fast forwarded from conception through birth. (Admire the perfect creation of God). Watch one or more of these videos numerous times. With the conscious awareness of how miraculous your body was formed, start believing that just like you were formed from an amazing intelligent Creator, that your body will always have the ability to regenerate and heal itself. The key is, to give it everything it needs to do this. This one is my favorite: *The Miracle of Human Creation* on YouTube: (https://www.youtube.com/watch?v=mCbS2ybYvUc). Write the titles/links of other ones you find below.

| |
| |
| |
| |
| |
| |

How did these videos shift your perception of your body?

| |
| |
| |
| |

Grow Your Own Garden

Think of your body as a beloved garden. Choose the flowers you want to grow. Plant the seeds. Provide nourishing soil. Fertilize it. Water it. Refrain from giving it pesticides. Feel the joy of seeing new flowers grow. Bask in the wonder of how much beauty can sprout from tiny seeds. It takes time for flowers to grow. Be patient with yourself as you nurture your inner garden and wait for your flowers to bloom.

After your flowers bloom, the butterflies will come. Remember that they were once homely caterpillars. In order to become butterflies they had to weave a protective cocoon around themselves. When you begin this journey, think of yourself as being in a cocoon, soon to discover you will become a beautiful butterfly.

It is also known that the reason gardening is so healthy, is because you are connecting to the earth. Most of us live on concrete and asphalt, and our shoes no longer have leather soles, therefore losing this vital connection. It is easy to forget that our Earth is a source of nourishment in more ways than just providing food. The earth, like everything else, is energy… energy we are meant to interconnect with. I once traveled to Muir Woods and stood inside a huge hollow redwood tree. The energy I felt was amazing, and I did not want to leave. I also noticed that when I hiked through wooded areas, I felt less pain and had increased stamina.

Choose the Flowers You Want to Grow

Sift through some magazines and find pictures of flowers to cut out and past onto page 9. If you would rather paint or draw, do this instead. Or take your own photos of your favorite flowers. You can cut the flowers out of these photos. By each flower, write a word representing something you wish to grow such as LOVE, JOY, GRATITUDE, HAPPINESS, SAFETY, SECURITY, PEACE, COURAGE COMPANIONSHIP, SUCCESS, CONFIDENCE, etc. Include one or more butterflies. The back side is blank to accommodate paint or glue.

Notes

List of what I would like to grow in my life.

My Flower Garden

Plant Good Seeds

Imagine that your thoughts are like seeds. Begin to write down the thoughts that enter your mind. Will they sprout flowers or weeds? When you spot a negative thought, respond to it as if you were talking to a good friend – tell yourself it isn't true and why. Then form a new thought that is closer to reality. Some examples are shown below.

WEEDS	FLOWERS
I am a failure at everything.	I am not always successful, but I learn something new every time I try.
I will never feel better.	Even though I feel terrible right now, I will not always feel this way.

Dr. David D. Burns wrote in *Feeling Good, The New Mood Therapy*, ten forms of twisted thinking. I recommend that you read this book and do the exercises in it. I have included brief descriptions after each one. After you read the list below, review the list of thoughts you wrote in the WEEDS column on the previous page. I don't know about you, but I was doing ALL OF THEM.

1. All or nothing thinking: (seeing things as either black or white, good or bad)
2. Overgeneralization: (seeing a single negative event as a never-ending pattern of defeat)
3. Mental filter: (picking out a single negative detail and dwelling on it exclusively so that your vision of all of reality becomes darkened)
4. Discounting the positive (rejecting positive experiences by insisting they don't count)
5. Jumping to conclusions (you interpret things negatively when there are no facts to support your conclusion)
6. Magnification (exaggerating the importance of your problems and shortcomings)
7. Emotional reasoning (assuming your negative emotions reflect the way things really are)
8. "Should statements" (telling yourself that things SHOULD be the way you hoped or expected them to be)
9. Labeling (the extreme of all or nothing thinking)
10. Personalization and blame (holding yourself responsible for events that are not entirely under your control or doing the opposite and blaming other people or circumstances for your problems)

Brene' Brown states that *"shame needs three things to grow exponentially: secrecy, silence, and judgment. Shame is highly correlated with addiction, depression, eating disorders, bullying... whereas guilt is inversely correlated with those things. People who are able to change their self-talk have better outcomes."* Are you beating yourself up internally with your self-talk? Are you your own worst enemy? Isn't it time you became your own best friend?

Dr. Masaru Emoto explored the theory that water could react to positive thoughts and words, and that polluted water could be cleaned through prayer and positive visualization. Your body is made up of 50-75% water. What are you saying to it?

Coach Laura Harris started a program for teenage girls called Power Girls. One of the things she talks to the girls about is bullying – that the worst bully is what they tell themselves. When she told me this, I knew this to be true for me. What about you?

Provide Nourishing Soil

You are what you eat. I am sure you have read this expression and heard it millions of times but lacked the self-motivation to refrain from eating junk. Dr. Harry Lodge (*Younger Next Year*) says to quit eating crap! Maybe you have told yourself a little of this or that won't hurt. But what if you saw your body as your precious garden? Until I thought of my body as a garden, it was difficult for me to avoid eating the numerous desserts offered at the potlucks and socials I went to.

There are tons of books about eating healthy, so I am not going to write another one. Remember the video of how perfectly and miraculously you were formed?

Read labels! Would you put the stuff they put in processed food onto your flower garden? Would you sprinkle your flower garden with additives, preservatives, and sugar? Would you water your flowers with soda? Avoid MSG aka Monosodium Glutamate! Avoid artificial colors and flavors! Avoid artificial sugar! And especially, don't give it to your children!

Consider where your meat is coming from. Because there is such a huge demand for meat, animals are being bred to grow extremely fast with hormones, are being given antibiotics to keep them from dying off, and they are fed GMO corn and soy. Most of your milk is coming from these same animals. What's more, with my Jewish heritage, I had learned that we were only supposed to eat "Kosher Meat" from animals that had been slaughtered in a compassionate way, so they do not fear or feel the pain of death. Can you imagine being one of those cows or chickens who has to watch all their friends and family members get slaughtered? Have you felt what stress does to you when cortisol is continuously released into your system? Have you or do you know someone who has had to fight in a major war and watched your buddies get blown up and killed? Same thing! Develop compassion for the animals as well as yourself! Watch the movie *Vegucated*.

Think about what you would use in a compost to add to your garden. These are the kinds of ingredients you want to put in your body.

Teal Swan has some great videos (YouTube) on happiness and self-love. In one of the videos she suggests that we ask ourselves, "What would someone who loves themselves do?" When I began asking myself this question, it became easier to avoid foods I knew were not good for me.

On the next page, list foods that are both nutritious and that you like. Create a master shopping list that is specifically for you (and hopefully your family) vs. using a generic one. You might also like to start cutting out pictures of these foods to create a collage of art. For me, out of sight is out of mind, so food art helps! Here is some space for you to glue or draw some food art.

My Shopping List

Fruit	Vegetables
Grains / Pseudo grains	**Nuts / Seeds**
Lean Meat / Fish	**Dairy (Grass-Fed) / Dairy Substitute**
Condiments / Supplements	Paper / Cleaning Products

Healthy Meals, Salads, Snacks, & Recipes

Fertilize

Fertilize your body, mind, and spirit with as much love and devotion that you would a flower garden. In order for your body to metabolize food, it needs vital nutrients such as enzymes, prebiotics/fiber, and probiotics. Without the above, food can become poisonous. We feel this poison as symptoms of pain, headaches, and fatigue. Then food can become toxic and turn your blood into a toxic mess.

Be aware that many food powders also have caffeine and caffeine type ingredients like guarana that can overstimulate your immune system. I myself, am super sensitive to caffeine so I stay clear of these. You may decide to start juicing. While I lived in California, I was able to get fresh carrot juice with wheatgrass in it almost every day for about $2 a glass.

Your body also needs oxygen and good blood circulation. That means you have to exercise (move) and breathe deeply. And hopefully, you don't smoke. I was the worst when it came to exercise and had lived a very sedentary lifestyle. Whenever I started a new exercise program, I would start too fast, burn out too quick, and quit. I had all those twisted thinking thoughts and convinced myself that I couldn't do anything. On top of that, I had fallen off a chair in 2005, and my legs got heavy and numb for many years. I had just found out that I had spondylolisthesis, so the anxiety and fear associated with my legs going to sleep had completely consumed me. I escaped major back surgery because my vertebrae were too porous to hold screws which turned out to be a blessing because I got the use of my legs back without it for about 10 years.

The book *Younger Next Year* changed my perception of exercise, with the theme being that it takes up to a year to get stronger (and younger), and no matter how old you are you are never too old to start. Dr. Henry S. Lodge (one of the authors) has seven rules:

1. Exercise six days a week for the rest of your life
2. Do serious aerobic exercise four days a week for the rest of your life
3. Do serious strength training, with weights, two days a week for the rest of your life
4. Spend less than you make
5. Quit eating crap! (you saw this one on a previous page)
6. Care
7. Connect and commit

Keep in mind, if you have a history of muscular skeletal issues like I do, you must start slow and find some type of movement you can do consistently. I started out with Curves after I found out the owner had overcome a bad car accident and ten surgeries through exercise. I knew if she could do it, I could, too! After about two years, I moved on to other exercise programs and purchased a recumbent stationary bike to use at home. Now I look forward to my exercise time as while the blood and increased oxygen is pumping through my body, the sensation of pain diminishes.

Our bodies, being energy, are also fertilized by sound. The Beach Boys got it right with "Good Vibrations." It is important to surround yourself with sound that balances your internal energies. One day, I had the opportunity to listen to various sizes of planet and crystal bowls being 'played' with a wand, I felt completely surrounded by the sound even though it was all coming from a single corner of the room. I then found a ten-hour Tibetan Singing Bowl Meditation on YouTube to listen to at home along with many other YouTube videos of various healing sounds.

You must also fertilize your mind, spirit, and soul. Find something you can believe in whether it is your religion or other spiritual practice. Meditate. Pray. Breathe deeply. Stop and smell the flowers. Read books about Positive Psychology. Watch inspiring videos (on YouTube).

Practice mindfulness. But instead of focusing on your ailments and all the things you have to do and are worried about, focus on how beautiful the drops of water are that you shower in. Refrain from working while you eat and focus on the taste and smell of the food. Appreciate the farmers who grow the food and all the people who took part in bringing it to you. Step outside and pay attention to the details of the trees, flowers, birds, and squirrels.

Write at least five emotions you want to FEEL every day (calm, content, connected, motivated) and ways you can achieve this.

How I Want to Feel:

HOW I WANT TO FEEL	WAYS I CAN ACHIEVE THIS
Inspired to get up in the morning.	Decide the night before one thing I would look forward to getting up for. Put sticky notes where I will see them when I wake up, like on the mirror over the bathroom sink.
Happiness	Watch YouTube videos of animals doing crazy things. Watch comedy movies and TV shows. Play with my cat. Smile at children and say hello to them.

Have a conversation with your pain or illness. You may be quite surprised by the answers that come to the questions you ask. I was. This is the conversation I had with my pain one day.

Physical Pain

Physical pain why are you there?
Taught to hold back, taught to beware.
Physical pain why so intense?
You live your life with too much suspense.
Physical pain why only inside?
Guilt you learned, true feelings you hide.
Physical pain what should I do?
Performing is what you should pursue.
Physical pain, what about love?
Let Spirit guide you, from inside, not above.
Physical pain, am I doing the right thing?
There is no wrong, accept what life brings.
Physical pain, will you ever go away?
Let go of this question, bless every new day.
Physical pain, is Serzone part of my life?
Worries like this will only cause you strife.
Physical pain, will you be there for all time?
Quit worrying, everything will be fine.

(I was taken off Serzone many years ago).

Conversation With My Body

Start a gratitude journal. Write at least five things you can be grateful for every day. After a while, this will become a habit.

Gratitude Journal

I am grateful for all the parts of my body that are still healthy and strong (and start listing them: my heart, my liver, my kidneys, etc.)
I am grateful for a warm place to live and a bed to sleep in.
I am grateful for nourishing food to eat and clean water to drink.

Find a cause bigger than your pain, illness, and/or depression to get involved in, even if all you do is answer their phone. Find some groups to join. Isolating yourself is one of the worst things you can do. Where I live, the Senior Center has a quilting group and a knitting group. A local church has a group that meets up one night a week for potluck and dominos. The Chamber of Commerce needs volunteers to help with events (or just answering their phone while they are out doing events). Seniors absolutely love to have fun! They sing together, dance together, laugh together, do crafts together, have meals together, etc. Even if you are not quite old enough (55 and up), you can participate in something they are doing together. You can even start your own group to meet in your home. I knew a lady in her 80's who had a group of musicians come to her house one night a week to jam. She was still playing an electric guitar! Meetup.com is a great way to start up a group. Start a book club or a philosophical group.

Groups I Can Get Involved In:

Refrain From Using Pesticides

Yes, pesticides. Bug killer. Poison. You do not want this on your vegetable garden because you know it is bad for you. You filter your water to avoid drinking toxic chemicals. You do not want to put it in your inner garden, either. Let the 'bugs' do their work.

Don't be so quick to medicate. Dr. John Bergman (my California family's chiropractor) wrote *How to Recover from Fibromyalgia*. Before John became a doctor, he had been hit by a speeding car that nearly killed him. His life was transformed by a doctor who told him that his body would heal and regenerate itself – but he had to believe this first. Among the topics covered in the book are diet, the alarming negative effects of the medications we (and I) have been taking to alleviate symptoms rather than treating the causes, and how our perceptions affect our outlook on life and on our health. Until I listened to Dr. Bergman's videos about our body's attempts to heal itself through the NATURAL process of inflammation, and that taking anti-inflammatory products do more harm than good, I didn't have a clue. Did you? I just accepted every prescription drug that was given to me, always needing one more drug to counter the side effects of the other ones.

I am telling you the following because it happened to me. Be cautious about taking antibiotics, which kill ALL the bacteria in your body, including the bacteria you need to digest your food and absorb nutrients. Most colds and illnesses are viruses which cannot be cured with antibiotics. Take antibiotics too often, and you are in danger of becoming antibiotic resistant and getting infected with systemic candida. Most doctors in the medical field don't even acknowledge candida as a reality, but it invades ALL the mucous membranes of your body, not just your vagina (if you a woman). If you keep getting recurring vaginal infections, you can pretty much assume candida has become a major problem. Once the invasion happens, it can take years to clear it out. It feeds off of sugar and simple carbs. Most people don't even realize what kind of monster/alien they are growing in their bodies. The same yeast that is put into bread to make it rise becomes a mortal enemy inside your body. Candida also affects your immune system so your white cells get confused and begin to attack the food you eat which results in major food sensitivities. Your immune system may even begin to attack one or more organs in your body. As I stated in the introduction, it took two years of restrictive diet and supplementation before I recovered. Then I thought I was immune to a reoccurrence and began eating junk again (which I stopped as soon as I realized my mistake).

And after I had taken hydrocodone (Norco) pills and muscle relaxers for 15 years to deal with pain, I found out from a neighbor about opioid-induced hyperalgesia. What a shock to find out! I am glad I stopped taking them before the opioid crisis hit and people were denied the pain relief they needed. I also found out that muscle relaxers can actually cause muscles to spasm.

On another note, fever is your body's way of fighting infection and dealing with numerous microscopic aliens that invade us. If you have contracted a virus, the only way to kill it is with fever. You just have to keep the fever below the 104/105 mark when brain damage might occur. Before you reach for the medication to reduce that fever, try placing a cool wet cloth on your pulse points (and the pulse points of your child), and for nasty nasal congestion, I found that a neck buddy you heat up in the microwave can do wonders to ease the discomfort. If you have a headache, try holding your hands over your face and head knowing that healing energy can flow through your hands. Ask someone in your family to do this for you, too. Try to save antibiotics for life threatening conditions.

Exercise will produce endorphins, your natural pain killer. When I could still walk, I used to have to go for multiple walks each day to get it flowing. Some other pain relief measures I have found are topical Lidoderm patches, a TENS unit, essential oils, and topical muscle ointments (without aspirin, and I prefer roll-on because it isn't as messy to apply). My favorites are Walmart's Equate Cool and Heat which has 16% menthol and Max-Freeze which has Ilex, Arnica, and Tea Tree Oil. They both dry up quickly and are less expensive than many of the other products being sold. It also feels great rolled onto my neck and chest when I feel like I am coming down with a cold or sore throat. Then of course, fertilize with healing sounds, Reiki, massage, hot baths, and showers, etc.

Don't poison your mind with negative thoughts. Refer back to fertilizing.

Water Your Flowers

If you have a garden (or indoor plants), you make sure to water them regularly except when it rains, otherwise they will wilt. The cells in your body are the petals and leaves of your flowers. You are 50-75% water. Your cells group together to intelligently form your organs, glands, skin, bone, muscles, ligaments, tendons, and the numerous paths and highways of your nerves and for blood flow. Watch the YouTube video again on how miraculously our bodies are formed. Your cells need WATERING – not soda and drinks with sugar, artificial sweeteners, artificial colors, and artificial flavors. I sincerely hope you reconsider what you are giving your children to drink as well as yourself. The difference here, though, is that the flowers of your body need watering a lot more often than once a day.

Dr. Bergman recommends drinking 50% of your weight in ounces. You can set a timer or an alarm on your cell phone to go off every hour unless you are good about drinking it all day long. Since plain water leaves me feeling thirsty, I found that adding an ounce of pure juice (like apple or grape) to it is like the spoonful of sugar that helps the medicine go down. Say a blessing over the water before you drink it (Dr. Emoto's way).

Try to get some water therapy. This can be hot showers, baths with Epsom salt, a heated swimming pool, a jacuzzi, and if you are fortunate, you have a huge tub that includes jacuzzi functions. There are devices that hook over the side of a tub to circulate water as well. I once went to a doctor of Chinese Medicine, and he prescribed these baths for me. Unfortunately, it was many years before I had the right bathtub to do this with.

You are asking yourself, "What would someone who loves themselves do?" Pamper yourself. Take the time for hot baths and showers. Take the time to give yourself a massage with your favorite lotion (unless you have a partner that can do this for you). Think about how miraculous it is that you have skin! If you have a bathtub and can get into one, add two cups of Epsom Salt to it and soak. If you take sit-down showers, add a cup of Epsom Salt to a dishpan to soak your feet in. Add "Epsom Salt" to your master shopping list and read more about the benefits this salt here:

http://www.saltworks.us/salt_info/epsom-uses-benefits.asp

Shower your flowers with colorful raindrops. While you color in the circles on the next page, visualize them as happy colorful cells flowing freely throughout your body carrying oxygen and other nutrients, miraculously birthing new cells and regenerating every part of who you are.

Also visualize white cells protecting you from harmful bacteria and viruses. Children who have been taught to visualize "Pac Man" eating cancer cells have recovered from cancer. I imagine scrubbing bubbles melting all the sludge out of my body.

Be creative and give the cells on the next page personality. Color them all different colors. Give them eyes, whiskers, and antennas. The back side is left blank to accommodate markers or felt pens.

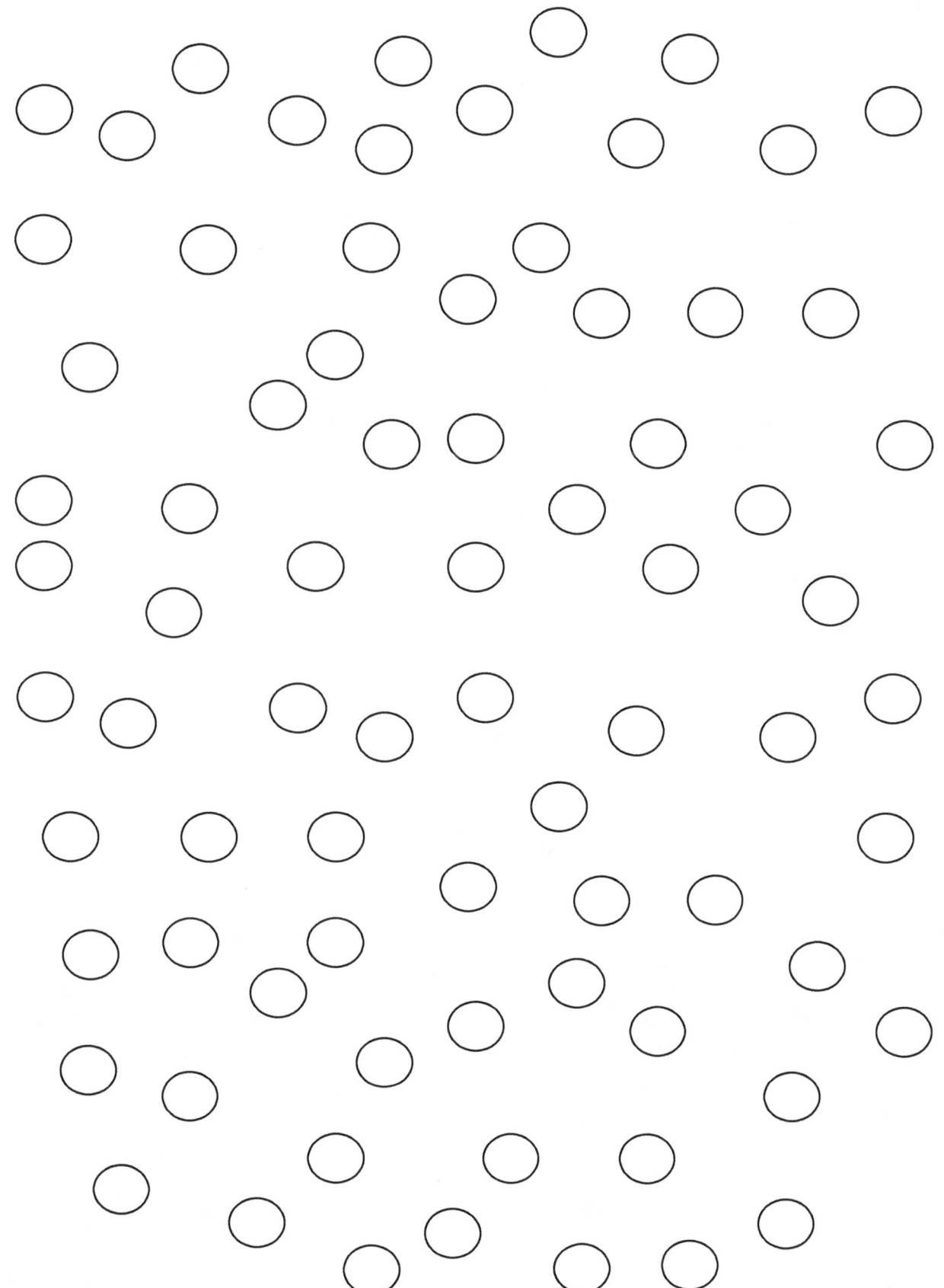

31

Feel the joy of seeing new flowers bloom,

and bask in the wonder of how much beauty

can sprout from tiny seeds.

Notes

List of things I can do to nurture myself.

What would someone who loves themselves do right now?

What are some of the steps I can take to make this happen?

Is there anyone in my life I am angry at or resentful toward? How is this affecting my peace of mind?

What traumas have I endured that I still affect me?

_____
_____
_____
_____
_____
_____
_____
_____
_____
_____
_____

What would I like to tell my much younger self?

_____
_____
_____
_____
_____
_____
_____
_____
_____
_____
_____

If I could do anything… and was given superpowers and a million dollars, what would I do?

Toxic things I can eliminate from my life (people, situations, food, junk, old clothes, cleaning products, soaps/shampoo/hairspray, deodorant, etc.)

What would I like my life to look like when I am 80?

How can my life experiences provide me with purpose?

Resources

American Academy of Pain Management (AAPM). For a comprehensive list of certified pain clinics in your area.
http://www.aapainmanage.org   209-533-9744

Goalistics Chronic Pain Management Program: an online interactive site that helps people with chronic pain to manage their pain and live richer, more effective lives:
http://pain.goalistics.com

Another online interactive site   http://painACTION.com

The American Chronic Pain Association (ACPA)
http://www.theacpa.org   800-533-3231

National Fibromyalgia & Chronic Pain Association (NfmCPA)
http://fmcpAware.org

National Fibromyalgia Association http://www.fmaware.org

United States Pain Foundation http://uspainfoundation.org

American Pain Association   http://www.painassociation.org

Self Help Treatment for Worry, Depression & Anxiety
http://www.anxietymadewell.com

The Mental Earth Community
http://mentalearth.com/index.html

Younger Next Year   http://www.youngernextyear.com

Reading List

Becoming Supernatural: Dr. Joe Dispenza

CFS Unravelled: Dan Neuffer

Feeling Good: The New Mood Therapy: David D. Burns, M.D.

Heal Your Pain Now: Joe Tatta, DPT, CNS

How To Be Sick: Toni Bernhard

How to Recover From Fibromyalgia: Dr. John Bergman

Managing Your Mind: Gillian Butler, Ph.D. & Tony Hope, M.D.

One Spirit Medicine: Alberto Villoldo, Ph.D.

Solving the Autoimmune Puzzle: Dr. Keesha Ewers

The Biology of Belief: Bruce H. Lipton, Ph.D.

The Body Keeps The Score: Bessel Van Der Kolk, M.D.

The Promise of Energy Psychology: David Feinstein, Donna Eden, and Gary Craig

The Truth About Chronic Pain Treatments: Cindy Perlin, LCSW

Transforming Anxiety: Doc Childre and Deborah Rozman, Ph.D.

Waking The Tiger: Healing Trauma: Peter A. Levine

Younger Next Year (for Women): Chris Crowley & Henry Lodge, M.D.

Other Books by Renee Alter

Appearances: A Journey of Self-Discovery

Reflections: A Toolbox of Poetry

Love, Life, & God: Getting Past the Pain

View From A Tree

Creating a Meaningful Life After Disability

Blog Therapy

Miracles Sandwiched Between the Challenges

Alternate Realities

Blogging a Path to the Future

Living With Symptomatic Spondylolisthesis

Lessons From Nature

On the Move

Metamorphosis

It is my sincere hope that this book has assisted you in growing your personal garden. Please leave a review on Amazon.

amazon.com/author/reneealter